Somatic Yoga Exercise: A Holistic Approach to Reduce Belly Fat, Stress Relief, and Weight Loss for Emotional Well-Being through Low-Impact Movement and Mind-Body Exercise

Florence E. Leiva

Disclaimer:

The information contained in this book is for general informational purposes only. The content is provided by (Florence E. Leiva) and while we endeavor to keep the information up to date and correct, we make no representations or warranties of any kind, express or implied, about the completeness, accuracy, reliability, suitability, or availability with respect to the book or the information, products, services, or related graphics contained in it for any purpose. Any reliance you place on such information is therefore strictly at your own risk.

About the author

Florence E. Leiva is a passionate advocate for health and self-development, devoted to helping people on their road to comprehensive well-being. As a prolific author, Florence has immersed herself in the areas of health and personal improvement, motivated by a deep-seated dedication to share information and encourage good change.

Married and anchored in the principles of family and connection, Florence gives a sympathetic and approachable viewpoint to her work. Her insights into the subtleties of health and self-development are not only influenced by significant study but also supplemented by her own experiences and the lessons learned on her life journey.

With a deep interest in understanding the secrets of human potential, Florence develops publications that serve as roadmaps for anyone striving to increase their physical, mental, and emotional health. Her publications integrate a broad grasp of health concepts with practical assistance, giving readers meaningful strategies to negotiate the difficulties of life and embrace transformational change.

Table of contents

Introduction

Finding a practice that helps us stay in the present moment is quite helpful in the busyness of contemporary life when our brains are constantly being tugged in different ways. In addition to providing a series of physical exercises, somatic yoga exercises cultivate a deep union of mind and muscle by re-establishing our connection with our body.

Describe Somatic Yoga Practices

Somatic yoga exercise is essentially a holistic method that integrates the integration of body, mind, and spirit rather than simply a set of positions. The Greek word "soma," which refers to the living body, is where the word "somatic" originates. It emphasizes the significance of feeling movement from the inside. By guiding us to explore the interior world of sensations, Somatic Yoga unlocks the possibility for significant change, in contrast to conventional techniques that may stress exterior aesthetics.

The Significance of the Mind-Body Link in Yoga

The body acts as a guide on the path to self-discovery. Somatic Yoga offers a place for introspection and self-discovery by acknowledging the inherent connection between our mental and physical states. With the use of helpful hints, concepts, and a wealth of information, this book seeks to walk you through the rich tapestry of Somatic Yoga Exercise and all the advantages it offers to those who take up this conscious practice.

Synopsis of the Work

We shall explore the history and philosophy of Somatic Yoga in the pages that follow, giving you a thorough grasp of its foundations. Helpful hints on how to do Somatic Yoga can empower novices and experts alike, promoting a secure and fulfilling practice.

We will examine the several advantages that transcend the material world and include improved self-awareness, emotional release, and mental clarity. The investigation proceeds into the domains of traditional Somatic Yoga, presenting its historical relevance and modern elucidations.

The core of our investigation, Somatic Yoga Exercises, will be revealed in a range of degrees of complexity so you may customize your practice to your requirements. We'll talk about how to incorporate Somatic Yoga into everyday life as a means of bridging the gap between the serenity of the yoga mat and the problems of the outside world.

We will provide resources for further study in the final chapters to inspire you to continue on this life-changing adventure outside of the printed word.

Join us as we explore the essence of Somatic Yoga Exercise, a practice that nourishes the body and uplifts the soul, bringing a deep feeling of well-being into all aspects of your life.

Chapter 1: Understanding Somatic Yoga Exercise

Somatic yoga: what is it?

"Yoga from the inside" is what somatic yoga is. Sensing your way into and out of the positions is the main emphasis. It is different from other forms of yoga in that it emphasizes the inside sensation of the poses rather than their external appearance. It is living in the now with kindness, awareness, and a keen sense of your body—all without pushing yourself, striving for perfection, or attempting to go there.

The Greek term "soma," which means "living body," suggests that there is a distinction between "the body" and "the living body."

A human being is just a body that has a certain form and size when seen from the outside. On the other hand, you are conscious of your thoughts, emotions, and goals when you look at yourself inside. You come to understand that you are more than just a physical being. Oma is your living, feeling, internalized vision of the world; it is what you feel and experience from the inside out.

The core of somatic yoga is exploration and emotion. We investigate motion and silence in a lighthearted but thoughtful manner. This kind and compassionate technique helps us rediscover our innocence and tenderness. This may assist you in

cultivating a more sympathetic connection with your body and yourself. These factors make somatic yoga an excellent kind of yoga for treating anxiety and depression.

Why It's Worth Trying Somatic Yoga

As you are undoubtedly aware if you have been following my work, I began experimenting around 4 years ago with incorporating several movement systems into my teaching and yoga practice.

I began along this new route because of the following observations that I made:
I feel entire and at ease when I am much more present within my body and let it direct my movements instead of relying on asanas or exterior form.
Like meditation, continuous micro-movements settle my mind and help me to live in the present now, but they also

do it more quickly, easily, and without causing me to feel tight or rigid in my body.
My body and mind experience profound levels of release, softness, and ease when I work with my body gently.
Movement exploration that doesn't rely on prescribed poses meets us where we are, and lets us release tension and emotion

helps us manage depression, alleviate anxiety, deal with grief, and reclaim our energy.

My nervous system is calmed and my emotions are under control when I approach my body with mindfulness and meditation.
I began taking lessons in Feldenkreis and Hanna somatics, two additional movement modalities, to include a more somatic approach into my yoga practice. These, along with my studies in modern dance, mindfulness, and relaxation therapy, were

all lovely compliments to my training in hatha, yin, and restorative yoga.

instructing in somatic yoga
Because of its conscious approach, somatic yoga, a more recent kind of yoga, is becoming more and more popular. Yoga and somatics, a movement discipline focused on how things feel from the inside out, are combined in somatic yoga. Thomas Hanna

created somatics during the 1970s. It helps remove ingrained, taught movement patterns that might cause pain by retraining the brain to enable muscles to completely relax and return to their natural condition.

The modern practice of yoga is all about doing what your instructor says, no matter how it feels. Most yoga instructors lead students toward the ideal alignment by teaching asanas (yoga postures) with precise definitions. You are encouraged by somatic

movement to investigate your feelings and use them to guide your movements. Putting your faith in your intuition and pushing yourself into a mold are two very different things.

By constantly experimenting with different ways of moving and being, somatic yoga empowers you to connect with your senses, and your authority, and move in a manner that feels good to you. Your practice starts to come from the inside out instead of the outside in.

You may develop a bond with your own body via somatic activities. They guide you toward embodiment, the understanding of and being in harmony with what the body is aware of.

Many individuals begin practicing yoga in faster-paced methods and eventually realize

it's not truly meeting their needs. People who desire to take care of themselves, really inhabit their bodies, and engage in internal self-care will find somatic yoga to be appealing.

Yoga: An Art of Somatic Movement
Although yoga is a somatic activity, it is often taught and done in a manner that prevents embodiment. Instead of being

aware of and feeling who we are, we are given instructions on how to move, which we subsequently "do" without experiencing.

A yoga instructor may provide instructions that have a "doing" aspect to them. A physical cue would encourage the pupil to explore their interests. A cue might take the form of a query or conjure up pictures. The somatic aspect of yoga emerges when we let go of the idea of "doing" and embrace a more experienced approach.

While doing an asana, you may want to consider asking yourself, "Am I comfortable?" Is your neck comfy when the instruction is to gaze up at your top hand? If not, are you able to get further assistance and make another decision?

Although there isn't much scientific study on somatic yoga, it's said to provide advantages such as reducing stress and anxiety, enhancing pain and injury, and assisting with hormone, sleep, and digestive problems.

Somatic Yoga for Emotional Well-Being

My instructor in my first yoga therapy class advised us to "work through the body when the disease is in the mind." Work with the mind while the illness is physical.

This has been confirmed for me in my work. Working with and through the body is very beneficial for students and clients who are struggling with mental health issues. This somatic method helps the mind untangle its intricate web of tangles. Then, we may rewire our brain and nervous system for safety, confidence, and resilience, and repair the tales from our past that are causing us distress.

A crucial component of somatic yoga is its ability to balance our neurological systems and enhance mental and emotional well-being. I like teaching yoga instructors how to include a more somatic approach in their teachings because of this. We teach how to become a therapeutic yoga teacher, teach yoga for mental health, and include a somatic approach into your lessons in our

one-year Somatic Teacher Training program.

Chapter 2: Mindful Awareness in Somatic Yoga

The Science Of Mind-Body Integration

The conscious experience and interpretation of physiological states and feelings is known as somatic awareness, and it is an important but sometimes disregarded component of health and wellness. It is a reflection of our capacity to perceive, decipher, and respond to physiological cues and is essential to maintaining a condition of equilibrium between the mind and body.

We examine the idea of somatic awareness, its advantages, methods for improving it, and the empirical data that backs up these assertions. As our knowledge of the mind-body link grows, there is great

potential to improve well-being and use somatic awareness as a therapeutic method.

Comprehending Somatic Awareness
The term "somatic awareness" describes our ability to consciously perceive and make sense of our internal and physical states. It's not only about identifying a feeling, like hunger or exhaustion; it's also about knowing what these feelings indicate about our general health and well-being.

One important aspect of the mind-body link is somatic awareness. It has been discovered to have an impact on several health outcomes, including the treatment of chronic pain. Gaining awareness of the signals sent by our bodies may help us improve both our physical and emotional well-being.

The insular cortex and anterior cingulate cortex are two key brain regions for somatic perception and self-awareness. These areas handle interoceptive data, or the perception of our body's physiological states. This clarifies the neural underpinnings of the enormous effects that developing somatic awareness may have on our health and well-being.

Mindfulness and Somatic Awareness

The concepts of somatic awareness and mindfulness are similar in that they both include paying careful, nonjudgmental attention to the present moment. Both are linked to better results for mental health as well as increased self-awareness and stress management.

Body scan meditation is one of the methods used in Jon Kabat-Zinn's well-known program, Mindfulness-Based Stress Reduction, to promote somatic awareness.

According to studies, MBSR improves interoceptive awareness, helps people manage their stress better, and improves their general well-being.

Techniques for Increasing Somatic Awareness

Body scan meditation is one of the simplest strategies to raise somatic awareness. This is a mental body scan where you tune in to your sensations without passing judgment on them.

Reflective Yoga

It has been shown that yoga, a kind of physical awareness combined with mental awareness, increases somatic awareness.

Practices that focus on alignment, breath, and feeling in each position help practitioners develop a closer relationship with their bodies.

Gradual Relaxation of the Muscles

Using this technique, one may increase their awareness of bodily sensations by tensing and then releasing various muscle groups. According to research, this technique may lessen anxiety and stress symptoms while also raising bodily awareness.

Body-Wise Perception

A therapy strategy called somatic experience aims to heal trauma by raising bodily awareness. Through this exercise, we may improve self-regulation, facilitate healing, and reestablish a connection with our body. Activities for Sensory-Motor Awareness

Methods like Feldenkrais, Alexander method, or mindful movement entail intentional and concentrated movements to enhance somatic awareness. These methods may increase one's awareness of physical sensations and boost general physical functioning.

Increased Somatic Awareness's Effects

Increased physical awareness may have major psychological advantages, according to research. It may lessen anxiety and depressive symptoms, enhance emotional control, and enhance psychological health in general.

Advantages for Physical Health

Significant advantages for physical health may also result from increased somatic awareness. Studies show that elevated somatic awareness is associated with reduced blood pressure, better sleep, and better general health outcomes.

Interpersonal Advantages

Improving somatic awareness may help in interpersonal communication and social interactions. We may increase our ability for empathy and understanding of others and promote deeper, healthier connections by increasing our awareness of our physical sensations and emotions.

Possible Difficulties and Misunderstandings

While there are many advantages to having greater somatic awareness, it's crucial to remember that excessive or too concentrated attention on body sensations may sometimes result in elevated tension or anxiety, which is often linked to somatic symptom disorders. The development of somatic awareness must be approached in an impartial, nonjudgmental manner.

Practices that improve somatic awareness often need the right guidance and oversight. Adverse consequences may result from improper techniques or a misunderstanding of the ideas behind these techniques. Thus, guaranteeing safe and successful practice may depend on the advice of qualified specialists.

In conclusion, cultivating somatic awareness may improve connections with others, improve mental and physical health, and generally improve well-being. Through engaging in mindfulness-based practices like progressive muscle relaxation, somatic experience, body scan meditation, mindful yoga, and sensory-motor awareness exercises, we may develop a deeper connection with our bodies and develop a more sophisticated understanding of how our bodies communicate.

The path to greater somatic awareness may present some difficulties, such as somatic hyperawareness, yet the advantages of this practice are many and solidly backed by research science. Future studies and methods may investigate somatic awareness in more detail and make better use of it as a means of achieving better health and wellness.

Chapter 3: Tips on How to Perform Somatic Yoga

ADVICE AND DIRECTIONS FOR SLOW SOMATIC YOGA

For people of all ages and capacities, Somatic Movement Flows® (SMFs) are all naturally safe. Because of this, their purpose is to reinforce and retrain the body's (Soma) brain-to-muscle memory. But, as with any new fitness regimen, please contact your healthcare provider if you have any physical difficulties or have any concerns.

SUGGESTIONS AND GUIDELINES

1. INTENT

Consciousness guides the path, and intention follows. Prioritizing your intentions will invigorate your practice and augment the advantages that come from your dedication to completeness.

The Sanskrit term yoga, which means "union," comes from the word yuj, which means "individual soul" or "self," and it also refers to the techniques used to achieve this oneness. Therefore, the primary goal of Gentle Somatic

In yoga, we accept and become one with our Soma, or Whole Self. This entails letting go of all judgment and accepting our bodies' seeming limits. It also entails letting go of things that no longer benefit us and loving ourselves.

A greater amount of room is made to awaken what is potential for ourselves on all levels when we let go of old habits and patterns of retaining tension in our bodies.

Our natural condition is contentment and tranquility. We were born with it. It is also among the numerous advantages of yoga that is gentle on the body.
"Make the difficult possible; simplify the feasible; elevate the simple."

2. GO IN A GLORIOUS WAY

Observe how your body responds to the Somatic Movement Flows (SMFs) and pay attention to it. If a certain movement in a sequence gives you a certain amount of pleasure, keep practicing it. Even while certain SMFs might seem difficult at first, they aren't supposed to be painful or taxing.

Never put up with pain. Pay attention to your body's signals and make the necessary adjustments. Respect the exploration process; comfort and movement will follow.

The "Three Second Rule" in Gentle Somatic Yoga explains how to prevent the Stretch

Reflex. A muscle group's automatic reaction to overextension is known as the "Stretch Reflex," which may cause a muscular spasm. In essence, this is how the body defends itself against harm. Say someone were to suddenly grab your arm; your natural reaction would be to retreat for your safety. See a muscle group acting similarly.

3. THE FEATHERING METHOD

Find your "edge" of pain while performing a movement sequence, and then take a little step back if you feel stiffness or soreness. With an eagerness to learn and a sense of wonder, carefully investigate the entrances and exits of space by:

Changing the angle's or vector's direction
Changing the motion's range and/or speed
Investigating minute motions by dissecting larger motions into smaller components

Every time you practice, slightly alter the instructions (e.g., changing direction or halting amid a movement).

4. SMOOTH AND SLOW

Developing an interior awareness of sensed sensation, or interoception, is the key to breaking old habitual patterns of retaining tension in the body. The area of your brain that gives you more mobility is stimulated by fluid, slow motions. Consider the Somatic Movement Flows as an exploration process rather than something to be hurried through. The finest learning occurs when the brain is at ease.

You are most likely suffering from sensory motor amnesia (SMA) if your smooth motions are broken up by jerking or skipping. This is a sign of good things to come—possibilities to retrain your muscles.

Either way, moving slowly and attentively will strengthen the activation of your brain's sensory-motor cortex. You will be able to move more freely and restore control over that specific muscle group by doing this.

5. Discovery Process

It is normal to feel confused while doing Gentle Somatic Yoga, even if you have been practicing for some time. It may seem like you are being asked to pat the top of your head and stroke your tummy at the same time!

A part of the science behind Gentle Somatic Yoga involves organizing the instructions and transmitting them via your body's movements. Determining the intricacy and specifics of a particular action helps a person recover from sensory motor amnesia (SMA).

Precision and coordination will develop gradually. And keep in mind that at GSY, creating anything "perfect" is not our goal. That isn't feasible! Enjoy the process of learning something new rather than concentrating on the result.

6. MOVE WITH YOUR EYES CLOSED

Through a process of neuromuscular reeducation, gentle somatic yoga enhances your awareness of your body from the inside out. Consider GSY as a kind of movement meditation.

It is best to shut your eyes and concentrate on your body's feelings as you practice your movements. Your attention could be diverted if your eyes are open, causing you to overlook the finer points of feeling.

Your brain-to-muscle repatterning will be more successful the fewer external stimuli you are exposed to. Soft lighting and soothing music—no TV, please—can have a relaxing impact that encourages more introspection.

7. "SECRET" TENSION

Selecting certain tiny muscle groups to repattern while keeping the rest of the body relaxed is part of the science underlying Gentle Somatic Yoga. Maintain your concentration on the precise muscle group you are taught to employ while maintaining a relaxed posture throughout to get the most benefits. For instance, if you are instructed to raise your left shoulder exclusively, do your hardest to maintain a neutral posture with your right shoulder, upper back, and legs.

8. The respiration

Generally speaking, no specific breathing pattern is the subject of Somatic Movement Flows exploration. The main reason is that there is already a lot to concentrate on since the majority of

SMFs include intricate and extensive instructions. The primary times

where this won't apply are during certain meditations, pranayama, and Core Energetics practices.

Keeping your breathing naturally flowing can help you develop an effective practice. Try taking a cleansing breath: inhale deeply with your nose, and then slowly exhale through your mouth while producing an audible "ah" sound. This will help if you find yourself breathing shallowly or even holding your breath. This will protect your body throughout the learning process and assist you in releasing any "secret tension" you may be carrying.

9. **REITERATION**

Three to five repetitions are typically performed for each set in a Somatic Movement Flow (SMF). Steer clear of excess; slow is preferable and little is more! Keep your attention on the muscles you want to repattern. Reeducating your mind and body (Soma) is what gentle somatic yoga is all about. As a result, before going on to the following Flow, give your brain some time to process the new information. As we've already discussed, the benefits are cumulative and build on the knowledge gained from earlier experiences.

Should you be recuperating from persistent discomfort resulting from accident or usage, you may think about doing SMFs many times a week.

You are free to investigate any particular SMF as much as you need to, at any time, if you are not healing from an injury.

10. **WORKOUTS ON A SOLID SURFACE**

Practice on a solid surface for optimal effects, to increase your awareness of the brain-muscle connection. It is best to lie on a yoga mat, blanket, or carpeted floor.

It's usually not a good idea to do the exercises in bed. The brain has fewer opportunities to absorb the information required for reeducation and repatterning on a surface that is too soft. But if you are bedridden, any movement, even little and deliberate ones, is better than none at all. One may also significantly increase the effect by picturing the motions (see the Miracle Moment SMF).

It is possible to adapt the majority of Somatic Movement Flows so that they may be executed while sitting in a chair.

11. **PUT ON COMFORTABLE, LOOSE WEAR.**

Throughout your Gentle Somatic Yoga practice, your body will move at different angles and in different directions. Wearing comfortable, loose-fitting attire, like what one may wear to a yoga class or the gym, will promote flexibility of movement without undue attention or constraint. It is advised that you take off your belts, earrings, and eyeglasses.

12. MODIFICATIONS AND PROPS Depending on your present degree of mobility, you may alter any of the somatic movement flows. Sustain an attitude of curiosity and discovery rather than result concentration.

Props such as chairs, blankets, yoga blocks, little cushions, and blankets may be useful additions that provide the ideal amount of support to boost your confidence and help you have a great practice. But don't rely on them as a crutch.

Even just picturing a Somatic Movement Flow may be very helpful for practitioners who have physical issues that limit their movement or cause persistent discomfort. It is feasible to start the process of restoring muscular control by envisioning an action before

executing it. This helps to create new neural pathways in the brain.

13. **Physical Exams**

The input you are receiving from each body scan is crucial to breaking old patterns of harboring tension and discomfort in your body, in addition to helping you feel at ease and content. Enjoy the fruits of your labor for a while!

Take a moment to process the new information and become aware of all the feelings that are emerging in your body after every Somatic Movement Flow. This should take at least sixty seconds. As you pay attention to your breathing, note your feelings. You become conscious of yourself as "witness consciousness" by doing this. As seen The state of being the Whole Self (Soma) is called consciousness.

Additionally, practitioners may experience a startling feeling of effervescence inside their Soma, which sometimes manifests as a faint buzzing sensation just under the skin. This seems to be a distinctive hallmark that comes from doing gentle somatic yoga. It's possible that this feeling is the consequence of more Prana, or life force energy, flowing freely throughout the Soma.

Chapter 4: Benefits of Somatic Yoga

One kind of exercise that people of any age may practice with ease is yoga. "Soma" means "body," and "somatic" describes the body's profound sensory experience. Somatic Movement There is a kind of yoga where you move with grace and awareness, focusing on your body and your breath.

This kind of yoga incorporates deep stretches, breathing exercises, and flowing sequences.

The following are only a few advantages:

joint lubrication and expanded range of motion

Somatic movement Yoga is similar to lightly oiling your joints. Your joints feel less tight and more flexible as a result of the deliberate and fluid motions that

encourage the natural fluids in them to flow. It's a gentle method to maintain your body's natural range of motion and, in time, may help improve joint health. Age-related changes in connective tissues, muscle stiffness, and joint wear all contribute to a reduction in range of motion.

Thus, by lubricating the joints, these exercises may aid in extending the body's range of motion.

Adaptability

A delicate dance for your body is what somatic flow yoga is like. The motions are linked and flowing, resulting in a continuous and easy flow. It's about moving with elegance and awareness, not about keeping rigid stances. This fluidity makes your body move more harmoniously, increases flexibility, and lessens stiffness.

endurance and stamina

Somatic flow yoga's fluid movements aid in increasing stamina, while attentive breathing practices enhance physical activity endurance. Regular practice may help you feel more energized and able to focus on tasks for extended periods. It's a subdued yet efficient method of gradually increasing stamina and endurance.

supple vertebrae

This exercise often includes core-strengthening exercises that stabilize the spine.

Frequent practice might result in a spine that is more flexible and strong.

improved health of the feet

Knee health depends on having healthy feet. Somatic exercises increase the strength and flexibility of the feet, which often improves knee stability.

enhances alignment of the body

Think of somatic yoga as your body's friendly coach. You learn how to move in a manner that is comfortable for you. similar to when you sit comfortably and stand tall due to better knee and foot stability.

Improved balance may be attained by regular practice, which will make daily motions seem more stable and under control.

Engaging in active meditation

Somatic flow resembles a serene, gestural meditation. It is similar to moving meditation as you go through the flow, focusing on your breathing and body.

In summary, this kind of practice leads to active meditation by enabling the body to access far greater levels of body knowledge, aliveness, and depth of present.

Physical Benefits

Regularly engaging in this kind of yoga may benefit you in many ways. You should be aware of the following health advantages of somatic yoga:

1. **Increases adaptability**

Somatic yoga uses soft, flowing poses that promote mobility, alleviate muscle tension, and develop flexibility. According to the experts, it improves general flexibility via deliberate motions.

2. **lessens tension**

Although stress is inevitable in daily life, somatic yoga practice may lessen its effects. This kind of yoga uses slow, deliberate movements to assist you de-stress and calm your mind. By incorporating this kind of yoga into your practice, you may help prevent stress and tension and help your mind relax.

3. Strengthens the body-mind connection

According to Kapoor, it fosters a stronger connection to physical experiences. This is because the practice's main goal is to cultivate awareness of one's own body—its movements, breath, and feelings.

4. Eases discomfort

Somatic yoga helps you release holding patterns in your muscles and move mindfully, which may help you get rid of chronic pain, particularly in places where tension and stress are present.

5. Corrects posture

This kind of yoga often includes awareness of posture and body alignment, which helps to improve posture generally. People who are more aware of their body's natural alignment may lower their risk of injury and chronic pain by incorporating this knowledge into their regular activities.

For whom is somatic yoga not advisable?
Even though somatic yoga is safe, those who have injuries or underlying medical conditions should see a doctor before beginning. Pay attention to your body and refrain from using excessive force.

But before doing this kind of yoga, expectant mothers and others with serious musculoskeletal problems should see a trained teacher or medical professional.

Chapter 5: Somatic Yoga Exercises

12 Powerful Somatic Rehabilitation Activities

The activities included here are a component of a therapy method known as somatic experience, which emphasizes intentional movement and heightened bodily awareness as a means of releasing trauma-related energy that has been trapped.

Somatic activities support trauma rehabilitation by using the profound relationship between the body and mind. These exercises combine the cerebral, physical, and emotional selves while calming the nervous system via deliberate movements and attention.

1. Grounding Techniques

One of the most effective somatic healing exercises is grounding. When unpleasant memories or worries surface, they help you stay grounded by re-establishing the connection between your body and mind via the activation of your senses.

Walking slowly, sensing the sensation of each stride, and feeling your feet contact the earth are a few examples.

Flowing warm or cold water over your hands, notice how the warmth makes you feel calmer.

giving yourself a gentle hug or covering yourself with a grounding sheet or soft blanket. They provide you with bodily comfort and help you feel connected to the energy of the Earth.

To absorb the energy of the Earth, use grounding mats or sheets that are connected to your home's electrical socket.

stroking a pet's fur and focusing on its texture and warmth.

squeezing a stress ball and focusing only on the force.

letting yourself be soothed by the tune of soothing music.

2. Illustration

By actively engaging with uplifting mental imagery, visualization is a proactive technique that may help you bring healing and peace to both your body and mind.

The Significance of Visualization

Visualization turns your mind into an effective therapeutic instrument. You may establish communication between your mental and bodily reactions by using constructive images.

By renegotiating events on a physiological level, this technique relieves disturbing images and creates an interior space that promotes healing and balance.

Examples of Visualizations

Imagine the first light of dawn illuminating every cell in your body and getting you ready for the day.

Imagine yourself in a calm, secure place where all anxiety disappears when things become tough.

Before going to bed, visualize the epitome of ease and relaxation to help you fall asleep and wake up feeling refreshed.

3. **The Body Scanner**

A great somatic healing activity to increase self-awareness and relaxation is the body scan. One way to become aware of and release tension or discomfort in your body is to slowly shift your focus to other parts of it.

I prefer to provide my customers with these body scan pointers:
Before you start, wiggle your toes a little. This makes your feet the center of attention. Next, slowly raise your attention, taking time to notice the sensations in each area of your body. Take your time.

Focus particularly on any regions that are tense or strained. Imagine the stress dissipating with every deep, slow breath you exhale.

Imagine a golden glow or warmth permeating your whole body to promote relaxation. How does that seem to you mentally?

The secret is to be kind to yourself and patient. Daily body scans for even five minutes may be very beneficial, but persistence is required. You'll get more adept at using this calming technique to release tension in your body and mind over time. Try it out!

4. Breathing Techniques

One of the most effective ways to feel focused and soothe the nervous system is to practice conscious breathing. Breathing

mindfully allows you to remain in the present moment rather than losing yourself in worry or emotion.

Here are some suggestions:

Imagine tension dissipating with each deep breath out. Breaths promote calmness and serenity.

Try box breathing: four counts of inhalation, four counts of holding the breath, and four counts of exhalation. How centering the equal intervals are!

To activate the diaphragm, try belly breathing. Put your hands there and inhale to feel it grow.

Breathing deeply has a great effect. Build up from 5 to 10 minutes a day at first. As you learn, have patience with yourself.

5. Techniques for Moving Your Body

Your body and mind may be harmonized via gentle exercise. It helps you feel more comfortable in your flesh by releasing pent-up stress.

Yoga poses that are therapeutic focus on the body. Move carefully, not brusquely.
Free dancing is a judgment-free method of expressing feelings. Allow your body to lead the way.
specific stretches for tense muscles. Breath and soft movement release tension.

Rolling your shoulders and neck may help release tension from stooping over desks and computers.
For 30 to 60 seconds, shake your body to release any trapped stress. (Although it may seem strange, it is helpful!)
Doing jogging or jumping jacks on the spot will help to regain energy.

During a walking meditation, you intentionally pay attention to every movement and feeling. Being outside brings tranquility.

Start slowly and concentrate on the sensation of the movement rather than the precise form. You'll gradually feel more integrated and balanced.

6. Securing With a Secure Touch

A caring method known as "containment with safe touch" employs tender physical

contact to engender a feeling of security and stability. It fosters a sense of internal

support and self-compassion as well as aids in the containment of strong emotions.

Examples of Containment With Safe Touch

Cradle your hands together in a gentle cup. Feel their comforting warmth as you draw

them up to the core of your heart and take deep breaths.

Give yourself a soft embrace and put a little pressure on your arms. Sense the rise and fall of your breath against the hug.
Place a cozy, weighted blanket over your chest or lap. Allow its soothing force to do its job, holding back challenging feelings.
Place your body where you are holding stress and lay down on a cushion or plush

animal. Its comforting softness may provide.

7. Materials

Resourcing is finding your sources of happiness, contentment, and fortitude. When things are chaotic, picture, recall, or use the things that support you:

Imagine a hug or supportive words from a loved one. How do they respond? Listen to their voices.

Picture your favorite place in nature. Enjoy the sights, sounds, and scents that make you feel at ease.

Play sentimental music that brings back happy memories. Allow the music to carry you away to a joyful moment.

Carry a motivational picture or item to help you stay focused on what matters. Allow its significance to serve as a grounding force.

8. Dilatoria

The oscillation between tense and relaxed states is known as pendulation. It promotes a greater comprehension and acceptance of one's emotions and behaviors by teaching the body to identify and value the difference between various physical and emotional states.

Methods For Applying Emotional Pendulation

Notice how each muscle group feels as you consciously contract and release it.

Throughout the day, rate your mood from 1 to 10. Observe how it flows and changes.

When you see yourself ruminating, take five deep breaths from your abdomen. Reestablish your core.

Take a stroll outdoors and see how your thoughts and emotions change.

9. Pulse-Inducing Motion

The body and mind may become deeply centered while engaging in rhythmic activities. In contrast to pendulation, which alternates between tensing and relaxing, rhythmic movement promotes a free-flowing descent into your body's natural rhythms.

These innate movements bring us into harmony with the internal rhythms we are all born with.

How to Perform Rhythmic Movement
Allow your body to softly swing from side to side or front to back, transforming into a natural, flowing dance.
To relieve stress in your spine, tilt your head forward and back while rocking your body.

To discover your natural rhythm, pick a leisurely walking speed and time your arm swings with each stride.
The secret is to tune into rhythms that feel pleasant in your body rather than forcing any movements. Make gentle, smooth, and intuitive movements.

The practice of bioenergetics teaches you how to manipulate your body's energy flow to improve your general health. Energetic obstructions result from our emotional states interfering with this flow.

Bioenergy: What Is It?

The vibration, heat, and current that animate your body's processes is known as bioenergy. Poor posture suppressed emotions, and long-term stress may all limit your bioenergy.

Exercise Ideas for Bioenergetics
Perform whole-body vibrations to release accumulated energy and relieve long-term stress.
To enhance energy flow and clear congestion from the torso, try doing long stretches.
To foster the efficient circulation of bioenergy, learn tai chi or qigong.

11. Techniques for Self-Regulation

Although self-awareness and regulation abilities are developed by all somatic exercises, several practices concentrate on enhancing emotional control and resilience.

Strategies for Self-Regulation That Enhance the Holistic Toolkit
To improve awareness and attention in the present moment, practice mindfulness meditation.

Practice breathing techniques to control your mood and reduce stress.
intentional relaxation of the neurological system via guided imagery.
Breathe gently in your abdomen to "rest and digest" instead of "fight or flight."
monitoring stimuli and reactions to identify patterns in response.

The secret is to learn how to handle life's ups and downs by being adaptable yet grounded. Self-control abilities enable you to roll with the punches.

12. **Employing The Voo Noise**

The vagus nerve is activated when you make a lengthy "voo" sound, which tells your body to relax. It's a basic but effective tool.
Take a seat comfortably, shut your eyes, and inhale deeply. Smoothly and slowly exhale, making the sound "voo." Allow

your body to reverberate with the vibrations.

Repeat many times, concentrating on the relaxing feelings.

When feeling overwhelmed or nervous, ground yourself by using the "voo" method.
If overstimulated, reduce stimuli.
Calm down and go to sleep.
Get out of the "flight or fight" mentality.

Try different vibration, duration, and volume settings until you discover the one that works best. This simple somatic practice may bring about calmness quite rapidly.

A Seven-Step Somatic Practice to Handle Triggers

I created this 7-step somatic exercise as part of my Wholehearted Path program to assist people in actively processing triggers and traumatic memories as they come up.

1. Pay attention to the areas of your body that hurt. Tightness in the stomach? clenched hands?
Breathe deeply ten times,
2. Increasing the force of your exhale to induce relaxation.
3. Think about a secure area. Imagine it clearly, utilizing every sensation in your body.

4. Permit movement that comes from your primitive, natural body and feels pleasant. Stomp, sway, and shake.

5. Go back to your anchor, the vision of your safe zone.
6. To activate your vagus nerve, make the "voo" sound while taking deep breaths out.
7. Give yourself comforting, kind words. Do you need to hear anything?

Repeat whenever unpleasant feelings or memories come to mind. You may retrain your nervous system reactions with practice.

Chapter 6: Yoga poses that heal your body and mind

Yoga is an excellent physical practice that improves body tone, flexibility, and relaxation. It is also an effective instrument for healing both physical and mental ailments in different sections of our body. Humans have a propensity to cling to our sorrows, difficulties, and negative experiences. If we're not cautious, these feelings have the potential to settle within our bodies, leading to worry and sadness. You may replicate a positive sensation and eliminate any bad energy by doing yoga.

Nevertheless, when it comes to healing, several yoga positions may ease your discomfort or even cure it. You may eliminate headaches, joint pain, tension, and a host of other issues by doing a series of yoga positions. However, which yoga positions guarantee success? Here are 13

therapeutic yoga positions that practitioners of all skill levels may attempt.

Little Pose

Often, all that is needed is a return to the fundamentals. One version that resembles a kid in the womb is called child position. It's also among the most popular postures for relaxing. Your belly should be virtually touching the mat while you sit on your heels with your knees slightly apart. Your hands need to be resting adjacent to your body or extended forward. Essentially, your belly should be between your forehead and your thighs.

Before assuming this posture, you may put a bolster in front of your legs to improve it even more and get the greatest results. Next, lower yourself into the posture so that you seem to be clutching the bolster. You will feel at ease and your whole being will be nourished by this stance.

Cat Cow in a Seat

The stance known as "seated cat-cow" requires a full range of motion for all spinal vertebrae. Since the stance is so soft, you shouldn't be concerned about injuring your spine. The purpose of the position is to let you feel at ease and as if your body has enough room to accommodate you. Place your hands on your knees and sit down on your mat, cross-legged. Until you feel as if your sitting bones are your foundation, maintain an upright posture.

As you bend forward with your chest and arch your back, begin to inhale. As you release the breath, round your back as if you're gazing down your navel. Carry out this exercise many times.

If you find it unpleasant to sit cross-legged, try bending your knees and keeping your feet off of your pelvis. Your hips should be just over your feet.

Pose for Constructive Rest

Do you experience back pain? As a passive posture that neutralizes your back and realigns your spine to reduce pain, a constructive rest pose can be the perfect solution for your back ache.

Laying on your back with your knees bent and your feet flat on the floor can help you into the posture. With your knees together, place your feet slightly wider than your hips. Relax your shoulders by placing your hands on your body. Take five to ten minutes to breathe in and out.

Climbing the Wall using your legs

Of all the restoration stances, legs up the wall are the most popular. The effects are felt throughout the body, starting from deep inside. All you need to do is locate a spot to sit where your rear end is closest to the wall. Your hands should be comfortably lying next to your body, and your legs should be stretched out along the wall. Make sure your body and legs are not overworked while you are in this posture. Take five to ten minutes to

breathe. After practicing this posture for some time, think about including leg variants such as bound angle legs, tree poses, and straddle splits.

Pose with Reclining Bound Angle

Restoring your body-mind connection is the first step toward recovery, particularly in cases of previous trauma. Posing in a reclining bound position enables you to see inward. Your body and mind explore interior feelings as you enter this yoga stance. You get more adept at identifying your feelings as you practice. As it strengthens the immune system and promotes the body's natural healing process, this position also helps with persistent colds.

Lie on your back to achieve a reclining bound angle stance. As much as you can, bend your knees and pull them up to

your pelvis. Let the soles of your feet contact as you extend your knees outward. To keep the

strain on the inner thighs from feeling too severe, place a bolster beneath each knee.

Put one hand behind your head and the other on your tummy, or rest them on the sides of your belly. Breathe consistently and gently for a minimum of five minutes.

Combatant II

Practice a Warrior II yoga stance to awaken your strength, ignite some fire in your legs, and open your heart. Pose therapy enhances blood circulation and breathing. Your body tones while you're in the stance. Legs, shoulders, and ankles are also strengthened. Maintaining this stance for longer than you tell yourself is the key to mastering it. Warrior II stimulates abdominal organs and eases

back discomfort by pushing you a little farther. If you too have knee discomfort, you should try this stance.

Dog Facing Downward and Using Foot Pedal

Do you wear heels and find that your ankles are sore or worn out? Would you want to make that right? To extend your feet and ankles and counterbalance the unnatural appearance of high heels, try a downward-facing dog yoga posture.

Stretch your legs behind you after starting on your hands and knees. Ideally, form a V-shape with your arms extended in front of your head and your torso, knees, and head all touching the floor. Make sure your feet are hip-width apart and your hands are shoulder-width apart. Use both feet to pedal for optimal outcomes. By transferring your weight from one leg to

the other, you may strengthen and extend each ankle.

Goddess Position

Once you lower yourself into position, you'll feel the heat in your glutes, despite how easy it seems. Those who operate mostly from a desk should apply for this role. Place your legs three feet apart as you stand. Once your thighs are parallel to the floor, lower yourself into a squat. You should never extend your knees beyond your toes. Raise your hands over your head in the attitude of prayer. Avoid bending or arching your back. For five deep breaths, hold the location.

Boat Position

For those who feel that their core is not as supportive, try boat posture. By using your body weight, this position helps you

maintain an upright posture and develop your core. With your legs straight out in front of you, take a seat on your mat. Press softly to the floor with your hands in line with your hips or slightly behind. Make sure

your fingers are pointing toward your legs. Remain seated and let your core become active. To create a 45-degree angle, lift your feet off the ground and point them toward the ceiling. Even better, spread them out even further so that your body forms a v. Hold the posture for ten to twenty seconds.

Grasping Position

Are you slouching forward all the time? Do your back and shoulders feel strained and worn out? Your upper back muscles may ultimately get strained from a

slouched posture. You may, however, counteract the impact, cure your back, and relieve the ache in your shoulders by doing the locust position. Additionally, this position will help you with posture and upper body tension reduction.

On a level surface, lie on your stomach. Stretch your legs to hip width and place your head on the mat. Open your hands and bring them to your hips. Lift your feet off the ground with the assistance of your hips. You need to hold up your head as well. You may extend your arms upwards or in the direction of your feet. Your upper back should ideally seem to be reaching toward your slightly elevated feet. As you breathe, hold this posture for thirty seconds. As you turn your left ear toward the mat, gradually release. Additionally, repeat in the right ear.

Pose in Bridge

Your neck will need to be saved after using your phone, laptop, or other digital device for most of the day. Fortunately, the bridge position may help you achieve your goals since it strengthens your back and securely stretches your neck. Place your feet level on

the ground and, while still lying on a flat surface, pull your knees towards you. It should seem as if you are about to do hip bridges. Ground your upper arm on the ground and extend it outward. Raise your torso and take five to ten slow, deep breaths.

Use a yoga block in the bum position if you think the pose is too difficult. It ought to support you in keeping your job.

Chapter 7: Integrating Somatic Yoga into Daily Life

Including Somatic Activities in Daily Life

It might be difficult to find times of peace and self-awareness amid the busyness of contemporary life. A powerful method to reestablish a connection with your body, lower stress levels, and improve general well-being is via somatic activities. While going to therapy sessions is important, including somatic activities in your everyday routine may increase the advantages and promote a more comprehensive healing process. Let's talk about how including somatic activities in your daily routine may help you feel more present, connected, and at peace with yourself.

Morning Intentional Breathing
Take a few minutes to concentrate on your breathing to start your day. Locate a peaceful area, take a comfortable seat, and shut your eyes. Breathe deeply through your nose, causing your belly to swell. Breathe out gently through your lips to let go of any tension or concerns. Continue doing this, letting each breath anchor you in the here and now.

Pauses for Mindful Movement

Throughout the day, take brief, focused movement breaks. Get up, stretch, and pay attention to your body's feelings. You may roll your shoulders, gently rotate your torso, or do a quick head-to-toe body scan. These bursts of activity may revitalize you and keep your body and mind from becoming stagnant.

Somatic Inspections

Before going to bed or during your lunch break, set aside a short period to do a somatic check-in. As you lay there

comfortably, mentally go over your whole body, from head to toe. Take note of any places that are tense, uncomfortable, or relaxed. Breathe into the tight spots and picture yourself letting go of any pent-up tension.

Conscientious Consumption

Turn eating into a sensual experience. Breathe deeply a few times and use all of your senses before eating. Take note of your food's flavors, textures, and colors. Chew gently and enjoy every taste, paying attention to how food feels on your tongue and body.

Relaxation Routine Before Bed

Before going to bed, practice somatic relaxation. Shut your eyes, lie down in bed, and inhale deeply a few times. Your head should be the last muscle group to relax after gradually tensing and releasing each

toe. As your body sinks into the mattress, welcome the sensation of peace that overtakes you.

It is not necessary for incorporating somatic activities into your daily routine to be difficult or time-consuming. By establishing a stronger connection between your body and mind, these simple yet effective practices may improve your overall well-being. You are nourishing your sense of presence and self-care when you welcome moments of mindfulness, breath awareness, and gentle movement. Keep in mind that

somatic activities are flexible, so adjust them to fit your schedule and tastes. As you progressively use these techniques, you'll discover that you can overcome obstacles in life and develop a long-lasting feeling of inner calm.

Somatic Yoga for Stressful Situations

This sequence draws inspiration from Bartenieff's Fundamentals, which emphasizes effective movement functioning and the intelligent use of breath, deep muscles, and core to enhance movement power and flow.

You may practice these patterns daily as a method to center and de-stress, or before and after your usual physical exercise since it's an easy movement. Practice in a quiet area, on the floor, or a mat. The most important thing is to

move gently and with complete concentrated concentration.
You might ask yourself, "Can I do this with 1% less tension?" and identify any body areas where you are carrying unneeded tension by moving slowly.

1 **Cross-references**.
Good for: discovering a soft core support; and establishing a connection with your psychological and physical center.

How to: stretch out like a large starfish on your back, arms, and legs apart. Feel the connection between your left and right limbs as well as your right and left arms. Visualize two diagonal lines crossing in the middle of your body, which represents your core. Press your right arm and left leg gently into the floor, then release your grip and let your arms and legs extend, hovering just an

inch above the ground. Repeat on the opposite side, being mindful of the two diagonal lines and moving carefully at all

times. When you return to stillness, observe how you feel after repeating each side five to ten times.

2. **Shifting positions**.

Excellent for: lengthening your whole body, increasing joint space, releasing tense shoulders and back, and teaching you how to gradually sequence movements over your entire body.

How to: As comfortably as possible, lie on your back in the same starfish posture. With as little effort as possible, move your left fingertips across your chest toward your right shoulder. Then, continue pushing through your fingers to reach for your right hand, gradually

rolling over to your right side. Keep all of your muscles as calm as possible and let your fingertips carry your whole body. After finishing the exercise, take a few deep breaths to relax, then roll

back to the beginning position. This time, start from your left toes and aim for your low diagonal on the left side, which is your initial position. Allow your head and arms to roll as passively as possible while you reposition yourself such that your left leg's energy is the only thing dragging you.

Repeat five times on each side, starting from the opposite side. As you practice, make an effort not to strain your lower backs; instead, softly hug your hips and ribs toward one another if you feel like you are about to enter a deep backbend or your back is hurting. Additionally, make an effort to constantly keep your

head on the floor so that you may get a wonderful massage and completely release any tension in your neck muscles.

3. **Bend your knee to form a fetal posture.**

Good for: relieving stress from your shoulders, back, and hips; experiencing your body's three dimensions, which may be missed if you just engage in very linear movement patterns (such as certain types of yoga or strength training).

How to do it: Lie on your back with your arms spread wide in a V shape, knees bent to the width of your hips, and the soles of your feet on the ground. Start by letting your knees sway and letting your body naturally fall to one side. Then, return to the center and repeat on the other side. Repeat a few more times,

letting your legs sink and relax. Continue into a soft fetal posture as soon as you are at ease. Drop your knees to your right side and raise your left arm over your head while keeping your fingers on the floor to lie comfortably on your right side. Feel

the little contraction in the center as your elbows, knees, head, and tailbone all move in closer proximity to one another. Swipe your left arm over your head and bring your shoulders back into equal alignment with the group to return to the beginning position. Let your knees and feet rock back to the center, making sure your toes are always in contact with the floor.

Repeat on the opposite side, letting go of all your body's weight and relaxing every muscle. Breathe in as you expand in your center and out as you draw

inwards on your side if that helps. After you return to stillness, repeat each side five to ten times, and then allow yourself some time to process the sensations.

Conclusion

As we come to the end of our journey through the field of Somatic Yoga Exercise, we are standing at the nexus of embodied knowledge and self-discovery. Our adventure has gone beyond the limitations of a conventional yoga practice, developing into a deep investigation of the mind-body connection—a dance that penetrates the complexities of everyday life as well as the mat.

A Tapestry Woven with Awareness: We are asked by Somatic Yoga to weave attentive awareness like a needle into the fabric of our lives. It is an invitation to completely live the present moment with an elevated feeling of awareness rather than

just a set of motions. Every breath we take and every motion we make on the canvas of our lives weaves a tapestry of self-discovery, intention, and present.

An Ongoing Voyage of Self-Exploration: As we get to the end of this voyage, it is crucial to understand that Somatic Yoga is a road rather than a destination; it is a journey that is always evolving and involves self-exploration. A lifetime dedication to fostering a harmonious connection between body and mind may be initiated with the help of the practices and ideas discussed in these pages.

The ability to alter oneself via the present is shown by the somatic yoga exercise. We may get a better knowledge of ourselves by opening the door to each moment with focused awareness. The body turns into a precious vessel that holds knowledge,

Taking the Practice Outside the Mat: Our investigation continues into the many occasions that comprise the fabric of our existence, not only when we fold up our yoga mats. It becomes a deliberate decision to commit to bringing the essence of the embodied present into our relationships, acts, and thoughts when we include Somatic Yoga into our everyday lives.

A Grateful Pause: As we conclude our trip, let us celebrate the beauty of conscious movement, the wisdom that lives within, and the body's resilience. Somatic yoga is a life-giving practice that leads us to a more balanced and harmonious way of living.

Acknowledgments and Closing Thoughts

Recognitions

We would like to express our sincere thanks to everyone who has helped along the way as we draw closer to our investigation into Somatic Yoga Exercise.

We are very grateful to the traditional yogic practices and trailblazing thinkers who have influenced the field of somatic movement. This book is built upon their knowledge, which is a tribute to the everlasting power of mind-body connection.

Thank you to all of the instructors and practitioners whose commitment to the practice of Somatic Yoga has enhanced the

content of these pages with their ideas and experiences. Others use your experiences and insights as beacons to help them on their life-changing journeys.

We are grateful to all of the readers and searchers who have joined us on this journey for their interest and candor. I hope that the thoughts on these pages speak to your personal experiences and help you develop a more conscious lifestyle with a stronger connection with your body.

Final Remarks

Let these words stick with you as we flip the last pages as a reminder that Somatic Yoga is a journey that extends beyond these words and is not a destination. Your body is the narrator in this ever-evolving narrative that is the practice.

I hope you apply the somatic yoga ideas to your everyday life and bring mindfulness to every moment. May you find a sanctuary—a place to explore, let go, and regenerate—in the silence between breaths and the soft rhythm of movement.

The practice of somatic yoga extends an invitation to enjoy the beauty of the physical present and to dance with life. May the vibrations of this exercise reverberate as you begin each new day, directing you toward a life of harmony, balance, and total well-being.

With appreciation and best wishes for the remainder of your trip,

(Florence E. Leiva)

Dear (Reader's)

I hope this message finds you well. We sincerely appreciate your support and the time you've invested in reading [Book Title]. Your insights and feedback are incredibly valuable to us.

As an author, constructive reviews not only provide encouragement but also offer essential guidance for improvement. We are eager to hear your thoughts on the book, from the storyline to the characters, and any other aspects that resonated with you.

Your honest review will not only assist us in refining our craft but will also help potential readers gain a better understanding of what to expect from [Book Title]. If you enjoyed the book, sharing your positive experiences can be a fantastic way to recommend it to others.

Feel free to express your thoughts openly, and if there are specific elements that stand out to you or areas where you believe we can improve, we're eager to hear those as well.

Thank you once again for choosing to explore [Book Title]. Your feedback is crucial, and we are grateful for your contribution to the literary journey.

Warm regards,

(Florence E. Leiva)

www.ingramcontent.com/pod-product-compliance
Lightning Source LLC
Chambersburg PA
CBHW070834260726
48660CB00005B/2046